Library of Congress Copyright Notice

Disclaimer

The information presented in this book is intended to serve as helpful guidelines only.

None of the procedures or methods taught in this book are intended to be used for diagnostic purposes: as always, it is your responsibility to only apply procedures which are within your legal scope of practice and you are competently trained to work with.

Masters In Massage Institute® and Dr. Koplen specifically disclaim all warranties, expressed or implied, for use of these materials, for any purposes, and in no event or use of these materials are they implying liability for results of its use.

Clinical performances mentioned or suggested are not claiming to represent indications or guarantees of anticipated future results. MastersInMassage® and Dr. Koplen do not guarantee any results or financial returns based on the information presented.

This system is sold with the understanding that the publisher is not engaged in rendering legal or other related professional service. If legal or other expert assistance is required the services of a competent professional person should be sought. All aspects of managing your clients' care must fall within you legal scope of practice and abide by regulations both legal and otherwise that are relevant to your practice locale and no information in this book should be used which may challenge or violate such regulations or laws.

Dr. Koplen specifically disclaims any liability, loss of risk, personal or otherwise, incurred as a consequence directly or indirectly of the use and application of any of the techniques or contents of this Course. Practitioners may use and benefit from this material differently and individual results will vary.

Learn more ways to advance your professional skills and practice success at MastersInMassage.com

Dedication

This book is dedicated to Massage Therapists like yourself who are committed to practicing with the highest professional standards and providing your clients' with the highest quality care.

You're dedicated to learning how to most effectively manage important aspects of your clients' care, which includes performing professional-grade examinations that help you assess what's wrong with them so you can provide the most appropriate treatment while effectively monitoring their care.

This book is dedicated to showing you how to do this.

Acknowledgment

My deepest appreciation goes out to the insightful and dedicated teachers and mentors who inspire and guide us along our educational journeys, without whom this book would not be possible.

Learn more ways to advance your professional skills and practice success at MastersInMassage.com

Table of Contents

Introduction 1

Six Tips for Keeping High Quality SOAP Notes 4

Subjective 5

How to Document What a Client Tells You 6

How to Accurately Inquire About Subjective Complaints 9

How to Measure Subjective Complaints 13

How to Write Subjective Complaints 19

Objective Findings 21

Four Objective Findings Found through ROM Testing 29

Why Significant Negative Findings are Important 30

How to Write Objective Findings 32

Assessment 34

How to Assess Clients' Follow-up Visits 37

Plan 42

How to Manage and Document Subsequent Client Visits During a Program of Care 46

Suggesting Self-Care Strategies 49

Learn more ways to advance your professional skills and practice success at MastersInMassage.com

Introduction

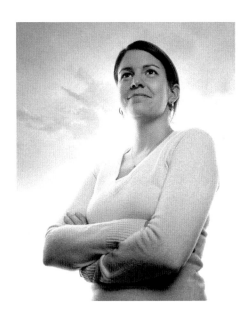

Most Massage Therapists agree that taking SOAP notes is the best, most professional way to practice. Yet many don't take them.

This is not surprising when you consider that massage schools do not teach this in their curriculum, at least not in detail, and most resources provide only superficial instruction for taking them.

Some MT's document findings that are specific to a particular technique they were taught, but not only does this fall short of mainstream-accepted standards, it also renders their interpretation uncertain when viewed by others and too weak to hold up to legal inquiry when requested for personal injury cases and other important situations.

Taking professional-quality SOAP notes essentially requires knowing how to gather the *right* information and artfully reduce it to properly-applied terms that are standardly used and understood by other health professions and practitioners.

It requires that you first have a fundamental understanding of *which* subjective complaints and objective findings to obtain. And knowing *how* to gather them, *measure* them, use this information to assess clients' situations, *plan* your treatments, and *monitor* their progress.

As the saying goes, it's somewhat simple but not easy. Unless you're shown how to properly do it.

Now you can relax and rest assured this course navigates you through the standard-accepted ways to take SOAP notes so you feel fully empowered with this skill-set!

Learn more ways to advance your professional skills and practice success at MastersInMassage.com

When several MT's asked me to provide a course that teaches you how to take professional-grade SOAP notes, I was initially reluctant without requiring that you first learn how to perform consultations and examinations so you'll know how to gather the foundational evidence that's used in SOAP notes. But fearing that if too many courses were required you may not learn *any* of them, a workaround approach was applied that takes key insights about subjective and objective evidence-gathering that are taught in my other courses (*How to Perform Professional Examinations and Consultations*) and succinctly blends them into this SOAP notes course.

Despite the brevity spent on these aspects, you can trust that this course still goes quite deep into showing you exactly how to take comprehensive SOAP notes.

Like most things in health care, SOAP notes don't need to be taken by "the letter of the law." Although it's okay for you to modify the full methods you'll be taught here to accommodate your personal practice style and shorten them as you desire, you're also encouraged to study them just as they're presented so you have a more formal understanding of how it's done.

As you continue to study and practice implementing these SOAP notes protocols they become easier to apply and your confidence grows.

Not only will *you* feel proud of your heightened skills, but your *clients* will view you with greater respect and esteem!

The Acronym S.O.A.P. Stands for

S = Subjective

O = Objective

A = Assessment

P = Plan

Here's How SOAP Notes Help You Manage Your Clients' Care

Soap notes provide important information about your clients' care.

They are specific and concise written records that summarize key essential facts about a client's status which you can easily reference.

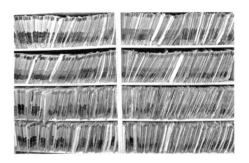

Soap notes help you form and define your clinical impressions and treatment plans for clients.

They allow you to document, measure and monitor each client's status and progress.

Not only are SOAP notes important for *your* own use, but other parties can access them if necessary, such as doctors, therapists, insurance personnel, and attorneys.

Learn more ways to advance your professional skills and practice success at MastersInMassage.com

Six Tips for Keeping High-Quality SOAP Notes

1. It's best to have **individual files for each client** and keep them well-organized and readily accessible.

2. SOAP notes ought to be **updated each time a client visits you**.

3. **Review a client's SOAP notes before each session** with you, even if it's only ones from their last visit with you, although it's often helpful to review them all.

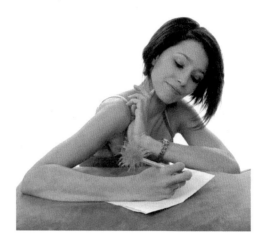

"A short pencil is better than a long memory."

4. **Write them down as soon as you** can because the longer you wait the greater the chance you may forget some information.

5. SOAP notes should be **written succinctly yet capture important information**.

6. They should be **clearly written and reasonably understandable**—at least explainable to other concerned parties. These notes are legal documents that may need to be used for medical, insurance, or legal purposes.

Let's Take a look at the SOAP Note Components and What They Each Mean

Subjective

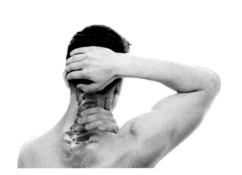

Definition

"Perceived only by the affected individual and not perceptible to the senses of another person."

Subjective complaints are "pains or problems" that a *client* feels or knows about, but typically not measurable by the examiner.

Examples of When and Where Subjective Findings are Discovered

New clients usually first express their subjective complaints, often referred to as "chief complaints," when filling out their Health History Intake form.

You can discover and discuss more information about their complaints during your initial Consultation time with them.

Although most complaints will be mentioned on clients' initial intake information and when consulting with them about their intake form information, they can be discovered at other times:

- Clients sometimes mention more subjective complaints during the examination. For example, a client may say, "I forgot to mention this but my neck pain often goes all the way into my shoulder and arm, which hurts when I try raising it too high."

- Subjective complaints are sometimes mentioned during the massage session. For example, while working on a client's feet they may tell you, "I forgot to mention this but my right foot has been causing much pain when I walk."

If a patient was referred to you by a doctor, their chief complaints may be written in the doctor's Massage Therapy Prescription request.

Learn more ways to advance your professional skills and practice success at MastersInMassage.com

How to Document Information that a Client Tells You

When a client tells you their complaints, here are two ways to document it:

One is to **quote what the client says**, if possible. By directly quoting what they tell you, you have an accurate description of their subjective complaints.

Another way, instead of quoting a client, is to **describe a reasonable interpretation of what they tell you**.

Either way, listen carefully to what they are *really* saying. Be prepared to "read between the lines."

Keep in mind that clients often misunderstand symptomatic rating systems, in which case they may need you to help them more accurately discern what's really going on with them.

For example, a client may say their back pain is a "10 out of 10" level pain, when what they really means is that their pain is mild to moderate most of the time, and at moments it becomes rather severe at say an 8 or 9, but it's not constantly that high.

You can clarify that a "10" is the level someone might feel when they get stabbed by a knife, shot, crush a bone, or give birth—in which case the client may adjust their rating to a 7 or 8 after hearing these comparisons.

Helpful Tip

When you gather subjective complaint information about clients, it's usually best to *not* question too deeply into *everything* that's bothering them.

Some clients have so many complaints, it's too overwhelming and time-consuming to discuss all of them. This especially applies to elderly clients.

Here's how to handle this: Focus your inquiry on a client's *significant* symptoms and complaints, otherwise known in the doctorly professions as their "chief complaints."

It's not that you want to always ignore seemingly petty complaints, such as a client complaining that their scalp itches when they wear a wool hat, but set your intention to ***focus on the important complaints* because these are the ones you will measure and monitor when gathering objective evidence**!

Learn more ways to advance your professional skills and practice success at MastersInMassage.com

Examples of Common Subjective Complaints

Physically and Neurologically Related Complaints

- **Tightness**
- Tension
- Spasm
- **Pain**
- Soreness
- Tenderness
- Burning sensation
- Numbness
- Weakness
- Other Abnormal Sensations ("paresthesias")
- **Painful or Limited Movement**
- **Postural Alignment Concerns**

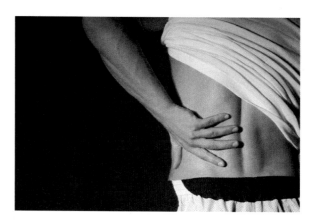

Emotional and Energetic-Related Complaints

- Fatigue
- Stress
- Emotional Disturbances:
  - » Sadness
  - » Grief
  - » Depression
  - » Worry, Anxiety
  - » Anger

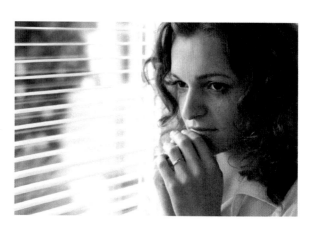

Learn more ways to advance your professional skills and practice success at MastersInMassage.com

How to Accurately Inquire About Subjective Complaints

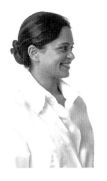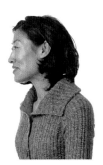

It's beyond the scope of this book to go into great depth about how to inquire about clients' chief complaints they mention in their health history intake forms, but you will be shown several important ways to accurately obtain and measure them.

Let's start by showing you how to address situations where clients may not clearly or explicitly tell you what their subjective complaints are.

It can be tempting for you to try to *guess* what a client's subjective complaints are based on the information they describe to you, especially when it involves stories about their life situation. But be careful when making your own assumptions about what they are telling you, because *your interpretation* of what's bothering a client may not be accurate.

To help you gather information more accurately, *specifically* ask clients if they are feeling or experiencing a particular subjective complaint.

For example, a client may tell you she recently went through severe life transitions, left an abusive relationship, and quit her job.

To verify her complaints, your best approach is to ask follow-up questions:

  ▶ *"How are you feeling because of your situation?"*

  ▶ *"How does this specifically bother or affect you?"*

Learn more ways to advance your professional skills and practice success at MastersInMassage.com

If a client has difficulty describing an emotion or complaint, it may be helpful to directly ask them about it:

> ▶ *"It sounds like you may be feeling sad, lonely, anxious, or angry? Is that true?"*

> ▶ *"Are you feeling tense, stressed, or possibly sore from all of this?"*

It's not common for their subjective experiences to be surprisingly different from what you perceive or imagine them to be.

For example, this seemingly depressed and fatigued woman may tell you:

> ▶ *"Am I feeling sad and lonely? Are you kidding? I settled my divorce from an abusive spouse and feel excited. I have a new job and a wonderful new relationship. I feel good—just somewhat stressed and sore from all the changes—and want to relax and celebrate my new life with a massage!"*

Here's another example of an indirect subjective complaint:

A client tells you:

> ▶ *"I've been working 75 hours a week at my job and have to continue until we finish an important project."*

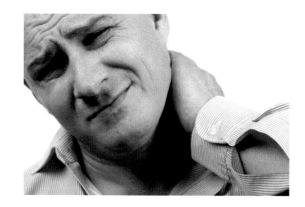

Notice how this client did not directly complain of (c/o) tension, fatigue, soreness, anxiety, or other symptoms. Although it's reasonable to assume the client feels some of these symptoms because of their stressful work situation, it's still the proper protocol to ask them if they are feeling these or other symptoms.

Clients Usually present with Two Types of Subjective Complaints:

One is more *physical*, such as **pain, muscle tightness, painful or limited mobility**.

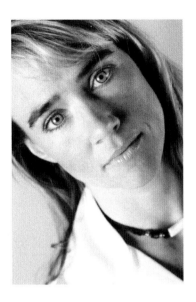

The other is more **emotional or energy related**, such as stress, depression, anxiety, fatigue.

(You'll soon be shown how to rate or measure each type.)

Nonetheless, you're encouraged to have clients relate emotional or energy-related complaints to physical areas!

By having clients associate their emotional or energy-related complaints to *physical* areas of their body, this **gives you more physically-based objective evidence to work with that you can examine and palpate during your massage sessions**.

This allows you to play a more direct and influential role in measuring and monitoring their objective changes instead of relying only on their subjective feelings that they tell you.

This is important because it gives you strong evidence to justify your treatment recommendations and gives you the ability to play a more involved role in managing their care!

So, if a client only presents to you with complaints that are emotional or general in nature, and not physical, such as complaints of stress, anxiety, fatigue, or if they say they want massage for general relaxation, here are two things you can do:

1. Rate the subjective complaints they mention (you will be shown how to do this soon).

---

2. Have them relate their complaints to *physical* issues. Here's how you can do this:

    First, ask the client if they have noticed their emotional or energetic complaint causing any p*hysical* symptoms—name some examples for them, such as:

    » Muscle tension

    » Tenderness, Soreness, Pain

    » Difficult or painful ROM

Next, ask them specifically *where* they feel it.

If they say something like, "I feel tired all over," ask them if there are any *specific areas* that bother them most, where they feel most sore or tight?

Next, guide them to relate their subjective complaints to some sort of *relief* that they are hoping to get from their massage session(s) with you, such as:

    » Relaxation from muscle tension

    » Relief from tenderness, soreness, or pain

    » Improved Movement

For example, ask them:

▶ *"Gail, you're obviously experiencing a lot of stress and tension.*

What would you like to get out of this massage—how can massage help you— maybe by helping to relieve some of the muscle tension and soreness that's manifested in your (e.g., neck, lower back) from all of the stress you're under?"

Learn more ways to advance your professional skills and practice success at MastersInMassage.com

How to Measure a Client's Subjective Complaints

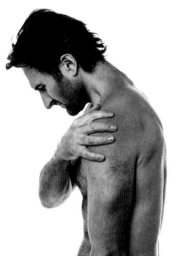

There are several systems that can be used to help qualify a client's subjective complaints by measuring or rating them.

Here are common ones that professional health practitioners use.

Three Important Measurements to Rate:

1. Severity

2. Frequency

3. Duration

Learn more ways to advance your professional skills and practice success at MastersInMassage.com

Severity

You can ask a client to describe (rate) the severity of their complaints from the following five choices. State all five for them, starting with minimum, so they understand the rating scale.

- **Minimum**

- **Mild**

- **Moderate**

- **Severe**

- **Extreme**

Another way to rate the severity uses three levels:

- **Mild**

- **Moderate**

- **Severe**

NOTE: For your personal note-keeping purposes, you can hasten writing this out by associating these words with numbers. This system is often used by practitioners as a quick, abbreviated way to document the severity of a client's complaints (and your objective findings which we will get to shortly).

- **Minimum = +1**

- **Mild = +2**

- **Moderate = +3**

- **Severe = +4**

- **Extreme = +5**

Numerical Pain Rating Scales are another common way to rate clients' subjective complaints:

1-10 Scale: 1= Minimum pain — 10 = Extreme pain

1-100 Scale: 1= Minimum pain — 100 = Extreme pain

After rating the severity, it's important to measure the frequency that a client experiences their complaints.

This is extremely valuable information to know that gives you important evidence when determining your treatment plans and for monitoring a client's progress.

Think about it: there's a huge difference between a client telling you they experience tension headaches constantly throughout the day, every day, versus experiencing them once a month, for a day or two, for a couple of hours a day, when trying to finish work-related deadlines.

There are many ways to measure the frequency of clients' complaints, such as how many days per week or month do they occur, which part of the day, etc.

Here's a Standard System used by Medical Evaluators to Determine the Frequency that Patients Experience Symptoms

Occasionally = approximately 25% of the time

Intermittently = approximately 50% of the time

Frequently = approximately 75% of the time

Constantly = approximately 90-100% of the time

NOTE: This is a more formal way of rating the frequency of occurrences and mostly used in workers comp or personal injury (PI) documentation, but it's important to understand how it works in case you want to use it.

The third thing to measure is the duration: how long does an occurrence last?

It can be measured in seconds, minutes, hours, days, etc.

The duration can sort of blend in with frequency.

What's important is for you to use these three criteria—severity, frequency, duration—for measuring or rating subjective complaints in *practical ways* that succinctly describe them.

Here are two examples of how severity, frequency, and duration work together:

1. Client complains of (c/o) *moderate* tension headaches in their sub-occipital area that occur *occasionally* at work, usually starting in the afternoons, two or three days a week. They last about two-three hours; more severe episodes last throughout the evening & she takes Advil for relief.

2. Client c/o of mod-severe (7/10) constant LBP past three days after heavy lifting. Last episode occurred 6 months ago w/ same symptoms (Sxs), relieved by massage and rest.

Another subjective measurement that's often used accounts for a client's ability to perform basic activities of daily living, which is technically referred to as "functional capabilities."

Activities of Daily Living (ADL's) which people perform includes any type of work and/or personal activities.

Oftentimes, work-related and Personal Injury ADL's are monitored separately from daily life activities, especially in workers comp or other legally regulated cases.

Measuring clients' capabilities to perform ADL's encompasses much more than just their subjective complaints: **It accounts for how their complaints noticeably affect their ability to *perform* various activities of daily living such as sleeping, exercising, housework, brushing teeth, cooking meals, sitting, standing, driving, doing laundry, sexual activity, and social activities**.

Charts that list common ADLs can be given to clients to rate their ability to perform various ones.

Charting ADLs is usually reserved for clients or patients who are being monitored in personal injury or work comp cases, although it's okay to use this method with clients if you wish to.

A huge benefit to having clients chart their improvements in ADL performances throughout their course of care with you is it allows you to measure and monitor these changes.

Here's perhaps the most practical way for you to apply ADL monitoring in your massage practice if you'd like to:

Find out what activity or hobby a client likes to participate in. Common ones include playing sports such as golf, tennis, bicycling, running, skiing, and team sports, and activities such as gardening.

Ask the client if and how their presenting complaints affect these activities.

For example, if they c/o moderate pain in their neck, shoulders, and arm, ask them if and how much this affects doing their favorite activity and make note of it.

Learn more ways to advance your professional skills and practice success at MastersInMassage.com

If they continue to see you for care and you continue to monitor changes in their subjective complaints, you can also *monitor improvements in their activity performance.*

Clients love to see how their massage sessions with you improve their sports activities, hobbies, and other important areas of their life—and make them more inclined to share their improvements with their friends and family and refer them to you!

NOTE: It's important to get a doctor's permission to monitor ADL's on patients who have been referred to you and you are both treating!

 Learn more ways to advance your professional skills and practice success at MastersInMassage.com

How to Write Subjective Complaints in Your SOAP Notes

As you've probably guessed, writing subjective complaints takes into account the important aspects that we've gone over.

You want to account for the client's important subjective complaints that they present to you with, such as pain, tension, limited mobility, or emotionally based issues.

You want to qualify things such as:

- How severe are their complaints?

- How often do they occur?

- When do they occur?

- How long do they last?

There are more questions you may want to ask a client, such as:

- What relieves your complaints?

- What aggravates them?

- Have you had this evaluated?

- By whom?

- What treatments have you tried?

- What were the results?

Learn more ways to advance your professional skills and practice success at MastersInMassage.com

Two Examples of How to Write a Client's Subjective Complaints

1. Clt. c/o constant +2 pain in left shoulder and neck, limited and painful ROM; pain is moderately worse when working. Started last week after water skiing, is mildly improving. "I can't work without taking aspirin every three hours. It's also hard to do things like lift my kids or reach for things overhead." Clt. rates constant pain 1-3/10 which increases to 4-6/10 during flareups. She also c/o feeling general stress and fatigue the past year.

2. Clt. c/o frequent moderate pain and tension in their lower back, occasionally radiating into their left gluts, slowly worsening over the past several weeks, aggravated by prolonged sitting. No injury reported but started hurting after gardening. Difficulty lifting, bending, and playing golf aggravates complaints.

 Learn more ways to advance your professional skills and practice success at MastersInMassage.com

Objective Findings

Objective Findings Definition

"Perceptible to the external senses; suggests an interest only in cold fact as distinct from belief, opinion, attitude, or sensations that are expressed subjectively by another person."

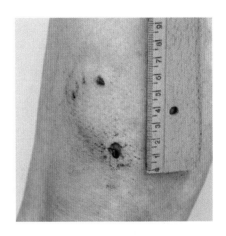

Objective findings are commonly found through various types of examinations and tests.

Simple yet important concept:

The objective findings that you explore and examine ought to be related to the client's presenting subjective complaints!

For example, if a client c/o pain and limited mobility in their right shoulder following an injury, you ought to examine that area first and foremost so your objective findings are associated with that area. In other words, it wouldn't be appropriate to examine their foot, knee, or lower back if their only complaint was their shoulder problem.

Arguably, you may perform certain types of examinations which indicate, for example, that a client's contralateral pelvic distortion contributes to their shoulder pain, or vice-versa. In such instances, it's best to examine *both* the focal area and the distant-related areas and be sure to qualify how the more distant areas affect their *specific* area of complaint.

Learn more ways to advance your professional skills and practice success at MastersInMassage.com

There are many types of "instruments" that can be used to detect and measure objective findings:

- Tape Measures

- Scales

- Goniometers

- Blood Pressure devices

- Stethoscopes

- Lab Tests

- Imaging Studies — X-ray, MRI, CT scan, PET scan, Ultrasound, etc.

- **Eyes**—Eyes can be used to visually INSPECT areas!

- **Fingers**—Fingers are considered instruments when used to palpate!

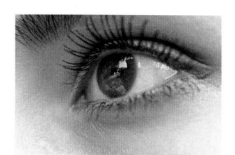

When you use your eyes and fingers to inspect, palpate, and facilitate tests such as ROM—or use other instruments you are trained to use—the findings that you gather are considered objective findings.

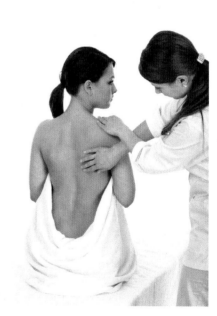

 Learn more ways to advance your professional skills and practice success at MastersInMassage.com

You will typically use any of these three exams to obtain your objective evidence:

1. Inspection

2. Palpation

3. Range of Motion Testing

Although it's beyond the scope of this book to teach you how to examine clients, we will describe the objective findings that you commonly find when you do examine them. (The book, *How to Perform Professional Examinations—Standard Protocols and Procedures for Massage Therapists*, teaches you how to perform top-quality examinations.)

IMPORTANT CONCEPT: There are usually only a *few* key objective findings that you need to concern yourself with that you will be looking for and monitoring when performing standard exams on your clients (aside from whatever findings you might obtain from performing an exam that's unique to a particular hands-on technique).

Common Objective Findings Found Through Inspection and Palpation

Abnormal Findings to Look For when Inspecting the Skin

- Texture
- Color
- Abrasions
- Moles and other lesions

Abnormal Findings when Examining the Skin and Myofascia

Inflammation

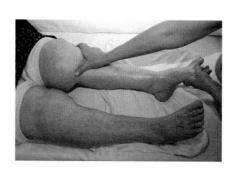

- The area often appears *red* (especially in the acute stage).
- The area often palpates as *swollen* and has a water balloon-like texture.
- Often *tender* to palpation.
- You may feel *increased temperature* (especially in the acute stage of injury).

Spasm

- An involuntary muscular contraction.
- Spasmed muscle contraction is usually temporary.
- Frequency, duration and intensity varies.
- Usually palpates as broadband muscle involvement.
- General soreness, usually w/o trigger points unless it's chronic.
- Spasm is often relieved by manual pressure, stretch, meds, and relaxation.

Hypertonicity

- Hypertonicity is an abnormal **sustained muscular contraction**.

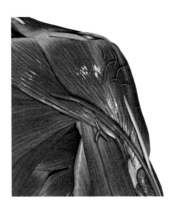

- Caused by abnormal neuromuscular involvement—usually CNS induced.

- Palpates as taut, wiry, cord-like hardened muscle fibers instead of a broadband texture.

- Painful focal muscle fibers.

- Pain often radiates.

- Focal inflammation may be present.

- Characterized by resistance to stretching unless neurological involvement is resolved.

Contractures

- Result from immobility, disuse, longstanding contractions and hypertonicity.

- If the inflammatory process develops it can precipitate fibrotic process.

- Less focal and less nodular than adhesions.

- Do not self-resolve and relax into normal tone and length.

- Moderately resistant to manual therapy and stretch.

- Proper directive force, pressure, and movement can help restore normal length and tone if neurological implications have been resolved.

Hypotonicity

- Abnormally soft or loose myofascial tone.

- Can imply muscle weakness, poor nerve supply to muscle, strain, disuse, subluxation, etc.

Important messages about managing TENDERNESS or PAIN that's elicited during palpation

You've surely experienced clients feeling tenderness or pain when an area is palpated, especially during a massage session, especially areas that are inflamed, hypertonic, adherent, or otherwise problematic.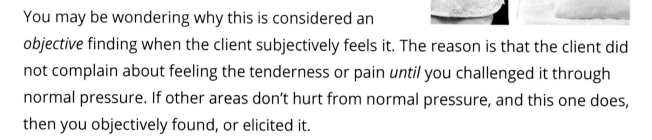

When pain or tenderness is elicited in a particular area when you palpate it with normal pressure, this is an indication that something is "wrong" and technically considered an *objective finding*.

You may be wondering why this is considered an *objective* finding when the client subjectively feels it. The reason is that the client did not complain about feeling the tenderness or pain *until* you challenged it through normal pressure. If other areas don't hurt from normal pressure, and this one does, then you objectively found, or elicited it.

Because tenderness elicited on standard palpation is a strong indicator of a "real and tangible" problem, it's important to inform clients to tell you if they feel any tenderness when you palpate them.

Tell the Client:

▶ *"Gordon, if you feel any pain or tenderness at any time while I am palpating you, I want you to tell me right away. Okay?"*

 Learn more ways to advance your professional skills and practice success at MastersInMassage.com

Helpful Tips

While palpating a client during your exam, it's important to palpate the area deeply or strongly enough to elicit a tenderness response, if, in fact, one exists. In other words, don't palate super lightly because you are afraid you might elicit tenderness in tissue that feels hard or tight to you. Obviously, don't use so much pressure that you *cause* pain or tenderness in an otherwise normal, healthy, non-tender area.

While palpating a client, ask them several times if they are feeling any pain or tenderness. This reminder is especially appropriate when you detect an area that palpates swollen, tight, restricted, lumpy, or hard.

Ask the Client:

▸ *"Is this tender to you as I press here?"*

If palpation elicits tenderness, ask questions that we previously mentioned to help you further evaluate your findings:

- What is the *severity* of the pain?
    - » Mild → Moderate → Severe?
- What is the *quality* of the pain?
    - » Sharp
    - » Dull
    - » Burning
    - » Tingling
    - » Numb-like
- Does the client feel pain *radiating* elsewhere?

Ask the Client:

▶ *"How tender does this feel—does it feel mild, moderate, or severe?*

▶ *"Is it a sharp pain, or just sore and tender?"*

▶ *"Do you feel tenderness anywhere else when I press here?"*

▶ *"Have you noticed this pain at other times?"*

    » *When?*

    » *How often do you feel it?*

    » *How long does it last?*

If tenderness or abnormal sensations are elicited during palpation, do the following:

• Note the specific *location* and if it *radiates*.

• Note the *severity* and *quality*.

• *Note any other important information* about this finding.

• *Document* your findings.

NOTE: If you don't want to interrupt the rhythm of your exam process by writing your findings as you go along, you can make a mental note of them and write them later in your SOAP notes. But it's best to jot them down at the time you discover them so you won't forget them.

Findings to look for when inspecting and palpating bone, skeleton, and posture:

• Abnormal *tenderness* elicited?

• Abnormal *location*?

• Abnormal *protuberances*, or *discontinuities*?

• Abnormal *asymmetries* or *deformities*?

Four Common Objective Findings Found through ROM Testing

1. Limited Mobility aka Hypomobility

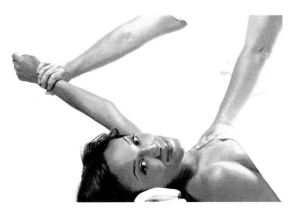

- Abnormally *decreased* ROM.

- Can imply muscle spasm, contractures, adhesions, sprain/strain, subluxation, intra-articular problem, pain, etc.

2. Abnormally Increased Mobility aka Hypermobility

- Abnormally increased ROM: this is a more rare finding than limited mobility.

- Can imply sprain/strain, ligament laxity, torn joint capsule, fracture, etc.

3. Painful Mobility

- Can be caused by any of the above-mentioned problems.

4. Abnormal Sounds: popping, shearing, grating, crepitus

- The word *crepitus* describes crackling, popping, grating type sounds that can occur in *any* joint and often heard in areas that are injured, inflamed, spasmed, degenerative, or adherent.

Learn more ways to advance your professional skills and practice success at MastersInMassage.com

When you come across positive ROM findings, document the following:

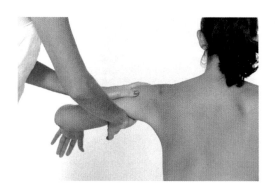

- *Which joint* is involved.

- What the finding is, such as *limited and/ or painful movement*.

- Which *directions* of movement are problematic.

- Note the *degrees* of movement.

- Note any important *bilateral comparisons*.

- Note any important *negative findings*.

IMPORTANT POINT: Significant negative findings can be important objective findings and should be documented in a client's SOAP notes.

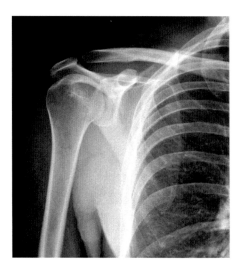

Discovering and noting significant *negative* findings, along with your positive findings, provides a more comprehensive perspective about a client's situation.

Discovering and stating negative exam findings also shows that you did, in fact, perform a certain exam or received other important information such as negative MRI or Xray findings, or other diagnostic findings determined by a doctor, which rule out certain concerns or conditions.

 Learn more ways to advance your professional skills and practice success at MastersInMassage.com

Three Examples of Negative Findings in SOAP Notes Documentation

1. Client c/o moderate pain when performing cervical Rt. Rotation and Rt. Lat. flexion, both limited to 45 degrees. No pain or limitation was reported on all other cerv ROMs.

2. A client recently fell and their arm is bruised, inflamed and very painful. You refer them out for further evaluation and X-rays rule out fracture. Ruling out fracture is a significant objective finding.

Client's bruised, inflamed and severely painful right arm-shoulder's X-ray report reveals no Fx or other noted pathologies.

3. Client's Rt side neck & shoulder region palpate with mod tension and elicit mild tenderness; Lt side same myofascial regions palpate normal.

Notice how providing relevant negative findings along with the positive ones provides a more comprehensive insight than otherwise would have been known from only presenting the positive findings.

Learn more ways to advance your professional skills and practice success at MastersInMassage.com

How to Write Your Objective Findings

Now that you know important objective findings to be aware of, let's look at some ways you can write them in your SOAP notes.

Terminology Commonly Used to *Describe* Objective Findings

The following examples are introductory lines that are standardly used to begin describing objective findings.

After you write an introductory line, you can continue to describe what the objective findings were. (Full-sentence examples are provided following this list.)

- "Inspection revealed…"
- "Upon visual inspection…"
- "Visual inspection revealed…"
- "Palpation revealed…"
- "Upon digital palpation…"
- "Digital palpation revealed…"
- "There was evidence of…"
- "There was apparent…"
- "There appeared to be…"
- "There were indications of…"
- "ROM testing results were…"
- "X-ray/MRI report stated…"

   Or simply state:

- "The findings upon (inspection, palpation, ROM) were as follows: _____."

Learn more ways to advance your professional skills and practice success at MastersInMassage.com

Five Full Sentence Objective Findings Examples

1. Inspection revealed moderately elevated musculature of the left shoulder, at the upper trapezius area.

2. Inspection revealed evidence of mild redness and apparent mild swelling at the area of client complaint. The upper left shoulder region appeared to be slightly elevated compared to the right shoulder, with indications of mild inflammation and muscle bunching detected upon digital palpation.

3. Palpation of the lower cervical region confirmed the presence of mild edema. Palpation further confirmed moderate paraspinal soft tissue muscular spasm & elicited mild to moderate tenderness response in this area. No other abnormalities or deformities were noted.

4. Palpation of the upper left shoulder area revealed evidence of mild swelling and muscle spasm. Right side palpated normal. Several TP's were identified, each eliciting a moderate pain response.

5. Cerv ROM tests: Lt LF & Rot 50% Nl [normal] w/ mod pain reported; other ROm's WNL. [within normal limits]

Learn more ways to advance your professional skills and practice success at MastersInMassage.com

Assessment

After gathering your subjective and objective findings, you're ready for the *assessment* part of your SOAP notes documentation.

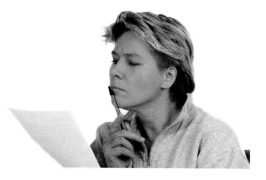

Assessments are your interpretations, clinical impressions, and formed opinions about a client's health status, especially focussing on their chief complaints and the subjective and objective findings related to them.

Your assessments attempt to piece together the information you've gathered to formulate your clinical impressions related to a client's chief complaints, subjective and objective findings, and in the case of established clients, their progress made from their care with you.

Simply said, your assessment is your succinct summation of what you believe is going on with a client based on the evidence you have.

While this may at first sound difficult or confusing, your assessment can often be stated fairly easy and briefly.

Keep in mind, you are *not* assessing clients for the purpose of diagnosing them—this is somewhat different.

On the other hand, if you want to make an assessment that gets more specific into *why* you believe a client's condition may exist (for example, ankle edema from sitting on a plane for 12 hours), or more etiological-based, or focuses more on assessments that are specific to a particular form of analysis that you've been taught, by all means, apply them. The methodology and examples that you're being shown here are not the only ways to determine and write your assessments, although they may adequately fulfill your assessment needs.

 Learn more ways to advance your professional skills and practice success at MastersInMassage.com

Sometimes your assessment can be as simple and straightforward as *correlating the client's subjective complaints with your objective findings*.

You can state, for example:

> The client's subjective complaints of week-long mild neck, shoulder, and upper back pain, and the objective findings of moderate muscle tightness noted and pain elicited upon palpation, and limited shoulder ROM in the involved area, all appear to be related to their recent water skiing over-exertion.

Notice how you did not state that you believe they have a sprain/strain, tendonitis, bursitis, or other pathology. You did not assign a diagnostic label.

You simply correlated how your objective findings appear to be related to their subjective complaints.

Another example might be a client who only complains of stress and wants massage for relaxation. You have them relate their complaint to specific body areas that bother them most and feel sore and tense, and when you examine these areas the muscles feel moderately tight with trigger point-like tenderness to palpation.

Your assessment could be:

> Moderate tightness and mod trigger point-like pain elicited on palpation to client's neck and shoulders correlates with client's c/o general stress with soreness and tension heightened in those regions.

Learn more ways to advance your professional skills and practice success at MastersInMassage.com

Your assessments include both initial assessments on new clients' conditions and assessments on established clients' progress and status.

As you read through the examples provided for you, it will make more sense.

Examples for Assessing a New Client's Condition

- Let's assume a client was recently involved in a whiplash type motor vehicle accident (MVA). The key to assessing this situation is to find out if their subjective complaints and objective findings correlate with one another and match with those that you would expect to see in a whiplash type injury.

- Do their subjective complaints—such as neck pain, stiffness, decreased and painful ROM, occasional headaches, and fatigue—seem to be the type of subjective complaints that would reasonably be expected to be seen in a client who recently experienced an MVA? Yes, they do.

- Next, do the objective findings you discovered when you examined them—such as mod-severely painful and spasmed cervical musculature, decreased and painful cervical ROM, and mild inflammation—seem like the type of objective findings that would correlate with their subjective complaints? Yes, they do.

- Do the combined subjective and objective findings seem like those that would be seen in a client who has recently experienced an MVA? Yes, they do.

If these findings all correlate with one another, your assessment can be written as:

Client's subjective complaints and objective findings appear to correlate with those that would be anticipated from this type of MVA and resulting injuries.

Learn more ways to advance your professional skills and practice success at MastersInMassage.com

How to Assess Clients' Follow-up Visits:

The key to assessing follow-up visits is to correlate changes in clients' subjective complaints with changes in objective findings.

What subjective and objective changes have occurred from their massage sessions with you?

- Subjectively, are their symptomatic chief complaints feeling better, worse, or the same?

- Objectively, what changes do you notice?

For Example, do improvements in their subjective changes, such as less pain and tightness, correlate with improvements in objective findings, such as reduced, spasm, tenderness to palpation, swelling?

If you are examining ROM, did you notice improvements?

NOTE: You do not need to describe the *exact* positive objective findings in *detail* when mentioning them in your assessments. It's sufficient that they are already recorded in more precise measurements or descriptions that can be referenced in the objective findings of your SOAP notes.

Learn more ways to advance your professional skills and practice success at MastersInMassage.com

Example

Client reports much decreased cervical tension, pain, and greater ROM. Palp revealed decreased spasm & tenderness. Increased cervical ROMs compared to initial exam 4 weeks ago. Client is improving from massage sessions.

Your Assessment should address why you believe the changes in a client's progress are occurring—for better, worse, or maybe no changes.

For Example

- Are they improving because of their massage sessions with you?

- Are they having a flareup because of an injury, increased activity levels, or stress factors?

- Is their condition *not* improving from massage?

   » Do you need to change your treatment approach?

   » Does their situation warrant being evaluated by a DC or MD?

Eight Examples of Written Assessments for Various Client Scenarios that May Present to You

1. A client reports feeling improvement and you notice the changes:

You can simply state:

> Client reports symptoms have decreased since last session – feels reduced tightness, swelling, and pain, and increased ROM.

> Muscles are mildly taught upon plantation and palpation still produces a mild pain response. Swelling decreased from +3 to +1. Cervical ROM is now WNL. Massage appears to be helping client's symptoms improve.

2. A client reports their neck and shoulder pain improved after their last session with you but feels worse this week because of high stress at work.

If the related muscles palpate more taught and inflamed to you than they did on their last visit, you can state:

> Client felt decreased tightness and pain for several days following her last massage, but work-related stress caused flaring with mild pain increase. Her neck and shoulders palpate moderately tight, inflamed and tender. Increased work stresses appear to have caused flareup.

3. A client is improving and reports feeling less pain and stiffness, and able to turn their neck better since their last massage session.

You might state:

Client feels decreased pain and tightness and increased ROM since last session. Palpation revealed decreased spasm and inflammatory swelling compared to last visit. ROM was within normal limits (WNL). Massage appears to be helping client's symptoms improve.

4. Example of a client c/o stress from working excessive hours:

Client's neck and shoulder tightness, dull pain, and accompanying exam findings of moderately taught muscles with mild inflammation and tenderness noted upon digital palpation, corresponds to their complaint of increased stress and tension from having to work excessive hours. No other unusual findings were found.

5. Example of a more extensive assessment describing a client's response to care:

Client responds well to massage sessions, reporting immediate decrease in symptoms after each session. Objective findings–muscle tightness, pain, and inflammation–reduce in intensity after receiving massage.

However, subjective complaints reportedly increase somewhat after two to three days following massage, presumably due to stress imposed by extra work demands causing flareups.

Recommended two massages per week to help alleviate flaring, but client cannot afford time off work and cost for this schedule, and wants one massage/week, which slows down progress.

Overall, massage is helping client to steadily improve from the effects of their MVA and life stresses despite intermittent flaring.

Learn more ways to advance your professional skills and practice success at MastersInMassage.com

6. Example of a client who has no specific chief complaints except feeling "stressed and fatigued."

Client reports massage is providing her much relaxation and helping to reduce her stress levels. Muscle tension and tenderness to palp in cervical region is noticeably decreasing.

7. Client reports postural alignment changes and decreased pain and tension.

Client states feeling her left shoulder and right pelvis returning to normal position with chronic moderate pain and tension in both areas decreasing to mild & occasionally no pain. Her shoulder alignment, neck protrusion, and high right iliac crest appeared close to normal alignment today & associated muscle tautness significantly decreased, indicating client is improving steadily from care.

8. Client's symptoms are not changing or worsening.

Fourth session in four weeks—client's neck pain and headaches are not improving; she reports mid increase in frequency, duration & severity.

Will treat today and monitor—if her condition does not change this week I recommended she seek evaluation from a doctor.

NOTE: The Masters in Massage book, *How to Professionally Refer Clients*, shows you the professional way to recommend and make client referrals to doctors.

Learn more ways to advance your professional skills and practice success at MastersInMassage.com

Plan

After writing your Assessment you are ready to write your PLAN.

Your Plan describes the plan of action you plan to take to treat a client and manage their care.

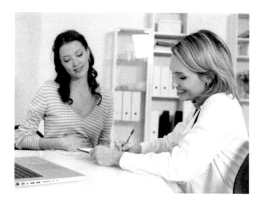

Your plans should be based on all clinical impressions derived from the important information you have gathered about a client.

Your plan for a client describes your treatment goals for addressing their chief complaints and other important needs.

Your plan may include other recommendations, such as suggesting self-care strategies, or recommending the client sees a doctor for further evaluation.

NOTE: In the event that you are working on a client who was referred by a doctor, the doctor may suggest chief complaint areas to focus on and specific treatment goals.

If they do not provide such recommendations, try speaking to them about this and discuss it with the client. This helps make sure everyone is in agreement, which is important to know especially if insurance reimbursement for the client's care is anticipated.

Learn more ways to advance your professional skills and practice success at MastersInMassage.com

Your Plan Should Include:

- **Will you massage the client or refer them out for further evaluation or other treatments?**

If a client's condition or findings warrant referring them out, it's important to determine which type of doctor or other specialists would be best. It's good to know the proper professional protocol for referring to an MD or a DC.

- **If you plan to provide a client with manual therapy, your plan includes your Goals and Intentions.**

  Examples
  - » Reduce Muscle Spasm
  - » Reduce Myofascial Contractures, Restrictions, Adhesions
  - » Reduce Pain
  - » Reduce Inflammation
  - » Increase ROM Capabilities
  - » Help Improve Postural Distortions
  - » Help Improve Client's ADL's at Home and/or Work.
  - » Provide Self-Care Strategies.

Important Message About Self-Care Strategies

When recommending self-care strategies to clients, be very careful to not violate what you are legally allowed to suggest or "prescribe." Laws vary state to state and even in municipalities in some states, but they typically do not allow MT's to make nutritional, exercise, or other health care related recommendations.

If you provide your clients with self-care strategies, mention them in your SOAP notes under PLAN.

More information about self-care strategies will be presented shortly.

- **The type of manual therapy or other modalities you plan to provide to fulfill your Goals and Intentions.**

  Examples of Manual Therapy Applications and Therapeutic Intentions

  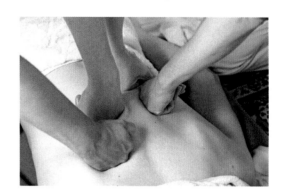

  » Cross Fiber Friction to help reduce contractures and adhesions.

  » Gentle Soothing touch to help client relieve emotional distress.

  » Trigger Point therapy to help reduce focal spasm and pain.

  » Petrissage to help reduce contractures and pain.

  » Swedish style strokes to help decrease spasm and pain, flush local inflammation, and improve restricted soft tissue mobility.

  » Manual Lymphatic Drainage to help flush inflammation.

  » Gentle stretching to help release restricted soft tissue movement and increase ROM.

  » PNF, MET, and AIS to help dispel holding patterns and increase mobility.

  » ROM movements.

  » Gentle traction to help relieve compression forces.

  » Muscle Spindle Facilitation to help stimulate weakened areas.

  » GTO receptor work to help release and relax taut areas.

  » Combinations of _____ to help improve structural alignment.

- **The Frequency, Length and Duration (number) of sessions.**

  » **Frequency** of Sessions: for example, 1x/week

  » **Length** of each Session: for example, 60 minutes

  » **Duration** of Course of Care: for example, 4 weeks

- Describe how you plan to Measure and Monitor the client's progress.

For example, by providing Progress Exams and Comparative Exams:

> Client to be monitored at each session; comparative exam at the end of 4 wk Program of Care with further recommendations at that time.

The Masters In Massage course, *Referrals and Retention Mastery*, teaches you how to create evidence-based programs of care where you measure and monitor clients' progress.

How to Write Your Plan

There are many ways to write your plan.

Here are some examples that show you how to write a plan at the *start* of a program of care and a basic plan *during* a program of care following re-evaluations.

Whatever style you use to write your plans, try to include all important information.

Plan for a Client Starting a Program of Care

Notice how this plan includes your **treatment intentions and goals, number of sessions** you recommend, and your **plans for monitoring progress**.

> Client is scheduled for one 60 minute session/week for 4 weeks to help reduce cervical spasm, pain, inflammation, and help improve ROM. Will provide Swedish connecting strokes, MFR, TPt Tx, & PNF. Recommend self-care stretching and cold applications to further help decrease inflammation, pain & spasticity. Will monitor progress per visit with Re-Evaluation in 4 Weeks.

How to Manage and Document Subsequent Client Visits During a Program of Care

5 Steps to Managing a Client's Subsequent Visits

1. Prepare for the client's visit.

Review their SOAP notes prior to their arrival. It's a good idea to review the chronology of *all* of their SOAP notes and not just ones from their last session.

Inform the client when they arrive that you want to spend a few moments to assess how they're doing.

2. Perform a Progress Re-exam.

Start by inquiring about changes in their SUBJECTIVE symptoms.

Ask the client:

- How have their areas of chief complaint, or other areas of significant concern that you've been working on, been feeling and/or functioning since you last saw them?

Note any improvements or lack of.

- If you happen to be working with a client who is also being treated by another practitioner, such as a DC, LAc., or PT for the same chief complaints, you may want to ask the client if they have noticed improvements related to *both* the other practitioner's treatments *and* yours.

Learn more ways to advance your professional skills and practice success at MastersInMassage.com

- Have their manual therapy session(s) with you been meeting their needs and providing them with what they were hoping to receive?

- Would they like any changes to be made in the treatment approaches you have been providing for them?

Note important information in your SOAP notes "Subjective."

Next, measure changes in OBJECTIVE findings and compare them with objective findings from their previous massage session(s).

Note important information in your SOAP notes "Objective."

3. If the client is completing a Program of Care, start thinking about the NEXT plan of action you will recommend.

4. Provide the client with a "Progress Reports of Findings."

Here's how to do it:

- Describe to the client—"report to them"—the progress they have made (improvements made) in their subjective complaints and objective findings. In other words, simply compare their *previous* or *initial* complaints and objective findings with their *current* ones: Tell them how each complaint's severity has decreased, relieved, or eliminated.

- Tell them the next "plan of action" you recommend for their next phase of care.

- If they are currently in a Program of Care, you can simply tell them you will *"See them at their next session, to continue keeping the healing momentum going."*

- If they are *concluding* a Program of Care, you can suggest the *next* Program of Care to them to help them continue to improve.

Learn more ways to advance your professional skills and practice success at MastersInMassage.com

5. Record this newly assessed information in your SOAP notes Assessment and Plan.

Example of your plan:

Client now scheduled for one 60 minute session every two weeks, for the next 6 weeks, to help continue reducing cervical tautness, tenderness, and to help further improve ROM. Will continue to provide Swedish connecting strokes, MFR, and PNF. Recommended self-care stretching, ROM movement and discontinue cold applications. Will monitor progress per visit; Comparative Evaluation in 6 Weeks.

Learn more ways to advance your professional skills and practice success at MastersInMassage.com

Suggesting Self-Care Strategies

When suggesting self-care strategies to clients, be sure to not violate what you are legally allowed to suggest or "prescribe" and knowledgeable about.

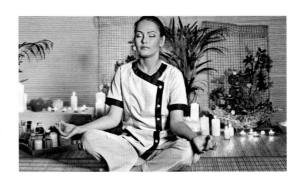

Although laws typically do not allow MT's to make many self-care recommendations, such as nutritional or exercise related ones, most MT's are aware of communications that you can use to suggest strategies which you are qualified to make, such as those involving stretching.

For example, you may tell a client:

▶ *"When my neck feels tight on the left, I stretch it to the right like this."*

Another example:

▶ *"Many people feel more energized, less fatigued and depressed, and even lose weight from cardiovascular exercises, such as _____.*
Have you considered this yourself?"

▶ *"Many people feel more energized, less fatigued, stressed and depressed when they meditate.*
Have you considered this yourself?"

Make sure the client understands your recommendations and instructions well.

When suggesting certain types of stretching, it's a good idea to demonstrate the stretches for the client, and if possible, have them perform them so you can critique them. It's always a good idea to hand them educational materials to keep that illustrate the recommendations.

Learn more ways to advance your professional skills and practice success at MastersInMassage.com

When the client returns for their next visit, ask them how they're doing with their self-care strategies.

If a client has confusion or complaints about a self-care strategy that another practitioner suggested to them, it's best to have them call the practitioner and explain the situation, rather than you giving them different advice which criticizes or overrides those instructions.

It's important to document the self-care strategies you suggest.

Common self-care strategies include:

- Exercise: Strengthening, Stretching, Cardiovascular, etc.
- Cold and/or Heat applications
- Postural and Ergonomic Awareness
- Nutritional and Herbal Related
- Stress Management Suggestions
- Proper Rest and Sleep

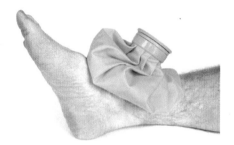

A popular self-care strategy mnemonic is having clients "take their MEDS"

M—Meditation & Mental Health

E—Exercise

D—Diet

S—Stress, Self Massage, Sleep, Sexual, Social Health

It should be obvious that when you write out your complete SOAP notes for a client simply write them in order starting with S and going to O to A to P.

Although it's a good idea to be succinct yet thorough while making sure you capture all important information, it doesn't really matter how long or short each category is.

For example, sometimes when doing re-evaluations on clients your assessment may be rather lengthy and your plan short. You may explain in detail why a client improves for short periods then experiences flareups, how they had an injury, perhaps saw other practitioners, is changing certain habits and self-care strategies … and why this affects their care with you … but your plan may simply say:

> ▶ *"Continue with current massage approaches 1X/week for 6 weeks then re-evaluate."*

On the other hand, your assessment and plan may be as brief as:

(A) Client continues to feel less stress, tension and soreness for many days following massage and overall decreased Sxs since starting care with me.

(P) Recommend continue with same Tx approaches and two sessions/month.

Notice how I simply circled the A and P and do the same for the S and O.

Use whatever style or system you like for writing your SOAP notes. I prefer lined paper that does *not* have the S O A P letters pre-written like some forms present because this lets me freely write each category as long or short as needed without being space-confined, then put the next one right below it.

Learn more ways to advance your professional skills and practice success at MastersInMassage.com

Your complete SOAP notes for a new client might look like this:

(S) Clt. c/o constant +2 pain in left shoulder and neck, limited and painful ROM; pain is moderately worse when working. Started last week after water skiing, is mildly improving. "I can't work without taking aspirin every three hours. It's also hard to do things like lift my kids or reach for things overhead." Clt. rates constant pain 1-3/10 which increases to 4-6/10 during flareups. She also c/o feeling general stress and fatigue the past year.

(O) Palpation of the upper left shoulder area and neck regions revealed evidence of mild swelling and muscle spasm. Right side palpated normal. Several TP's were identified, each eliciting a moderate pain response along traps to mid-back and deltoid to upper arm. Cerv ROM tests: Lt LF & Rot 50% Nl w/ mod pain reported; other serve ROm's WNL. Lt shoulder painful in flexion and abduction at 90 degrees.

(A) Client's subjective complaints and objective findings appear to correlate with those that would be anticipated from this type of activity/injury.

(P) Recommended one 60 minute session/week for 4 weeks to help reduce cervical–Lt shoulder/arm spasm, pain, inflammation, and help improve ROM. Will provide gentle Swedish connecting strokes, MFR, TPt Tx, & PNF. Recommend very gentle stretching and cold applications to further help decrease inflammation, pain & spasticity–client instructed to avoid pain in all activities. Will monitor progress per visit with Re-Evaluation in 4 Weeks.

 Learn more ways to advance your professional skills and practice success at MastersInMassage.com

Conclusion and Insights

Congratulations on taking your client management skills to a higher level by learning how to gather and document SOAP note information like a true professional.

Like any other knowledge or skills, it's important that you *continue to practice implementing and refining the methods* this course teaches you or any others you might use.

You're not expected to apply everything all at once but as you keep practicing implementing your new skills you will continue to feel more confident and be more competent at using them. Mastery requires practice and patience.

If you want to increase your client management skills further, look for other courses by Michael Koplen and Masters In Massage Institute on Amazon or at Mastersinmassage.com.

Learn more ways to advance your professional skills and practice success at MastersInMassage.com

About Michael Koplen

Michael Koplen, DC, MT, is an international teacher and National Chiropractor of the Year recipient through the prestigious Landis-Ward Practice Management group.

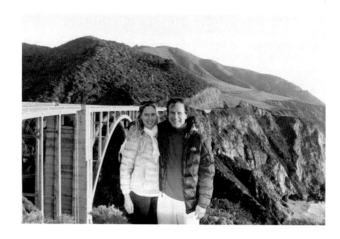

After completing the Boulder School of Massage Therapy he opened the innovative and highly successful Denver Massage Center were he practiced along with seven colleagues and taught massage classes.

Inspired to further his examination, assessment, and treatment skills, he graduated from Palmer-West Chiropractic College.

He is a certified Qualified Medical Evaluator (Q.M.E.) for the California Workmans Compensation system, a certified Personal Injury Whiplash and Motor Vehicle Accident (MVA) Evaluator, and served as a team doctor for the Cuervo International Beach Volleyball Tournament in Santa Cruz.

Michael founded the Masters In Massage Institute® and developed several courses for Massage Therapists to further advance their professional client management skills and practice success, which are available through home-study on Amazon and MastersInMasage.com and through live classes.

He currently practices part-time at the Capitola Health Center with two other doctors, three Massage Therapists, and an acupuncturist.

Other Valuable Courses to Advance Your Practice Skills and Success Found on Amazon and at MastersinMassage.com

How to Perform Professional Examinations – Standard Protocols and Procedures for Massage Therapists

Knowing how to perform professional-grade examinations on new clients is an extremely important skill to apply in *any* health care practice, including yours as a Massage Therapist.

This to-the-point book teaches you why it's important for you to provide standard exams similar to ones other health professionals use (in addition to ones you might apply for a particular technique's assessment), how it benefits you and your clients, and exactly how to perform them right away in your practice!

How to Treat Whiplash and Soft Tissue Injuries – Massage Therapy Approaches

This is an extremely important topic for Massage Therapists to become familiar with because whiplash and other sprain-strain type injuries are among the most common conditions clients and referred patients present to you with.

This course provides you with well-accepted soft tissue assessment and treatment skills that follow protocols Chiropractors and PT use, in practical ways that you can readily apply in your massage practice to increase your ability to confidently manage these injuries and make the care you provide for these clients more focused, effective, and reliable.

Integrative Care Mastery Course

Learn how to professionally manage clients and patients who also receive Chiropractic care. Comes with full video presentations.

Learn more ways to advance your professional skills and practice success at MastersInMassage.com

Referrals and Retention Mastery Course

Learn how to get high-quality client referrals without needing to advertise, recommend evidence-based programs of care to your clients so they see you multiple times, and easily recall clients who drift from care. Course comes with full video presentations that guide you through all important information.

The Chiropractic-Integrated Massage Practice

If you want to work in a Chiropractic clinic or alongside DC's and professionally co-manage patients' care, this course teaches you everything you need to know to feel fully competent and confident! Course comes with full video presentations that guide you through all important information.

How to Professionally Refer Clients

This straightforward how-to book teaches you how to professionally refer clients to doctors for evaluation when the need arises and make sure they return to you for further care. Comes with referral scripts, forms, and letters.

How to Connect with Doctors and Have Them Refer Patients to You

Let this power-packed 36-page manual show you the most effective ways to connect with doctors (especially DC's) and have them refer patients to you. Comes with time-tested strategies, scripted phrases, and a communication letter so you don't have to guess.

 Learn more ways to advance your professional skills and practice success at MastersInMassage.com

SOAP Notes Test Questions

1. **The acronym "SOAP" stands for "Subjective, Objective, Assessment, Pain."**

   True or False

2. **SOAP notes are confidential and HIPPA laws prevent outside parties such as attorneys or insurance personnel from requesting copies of them:**

   True or False

3. **SOAP notes provide a critical source of information about clients' care and should be kept by Manual Therapists.**

   True or False

4. **Which of the following is true about SOAP notes?**

   a. They should be updated each time a client visits you.

   b. Do not need to be taken seriously because they are never copied for medical, insurance or legal purposes.

   c. Should only be taken if your schedule allows enough time

5. **Subjective complaints are pains or problems the client feels or knows about and are not objectively measurable by the examiner.**

   True or False

6. **Subjective complaints may be discovered where?**

    a. In the client's Health History form

    b. Discussed during the Consultation

    c. Elicited during the Examination

    d. Described during the Massage Session

    e. All of the above

7. **It's advisable that when you gather subjective complaint information from clients, explore _everything_ that's possibly bothering them and dig deeply into it.**

    True or False

8. **Which of the following are typical subjective complaints clients present with:**

    a. Pain

    b. Limited ROM

    c. Stress

    d. All the above

Learn more ways to advance your professional skills and practice success at MastersInMassage.com

9. If a client's subjective complaints seem vague or unclear to you, it's best to:

    a. Respect their privacy and don't ask questions.

    b. Quote them and ask no more.

    c. Respect the "Don't ask, don't tell" policy.

    d. Ask questions to clarify what they are trying to convey.

10. If a client complains only of "stress" or "fatigue," it's best to:

    a. Immediately provide them with a relaxation massage.

    b. Guide them to relate their stress to physical symptoms in their body, such as soreness or tension.

    c. Suggest they take naps and medication.

    d. Tell them you're sorry they feel this way.

11. According to the notes, two ways to record a client's subjective complaints are:

    a. Just memorize it if you have a good memory.

    b. Describe a reasonable interpretation of what they told you.

    c. Make up what sounds good to you.

    d. Quote the client's own description.

    e. b and d

12. According to the notes, the three most important descriptions for pain occurrences are:

   a. Severity, Frequency, and Duration

   b. Severity, Frequency and Dependability

   c. Severity, Frequency, and Dependency

   d. None of the above

13. Which word for describing pain severity was not used in the notes:

   a. Moderate

   b. Super

   c. Mild

   d. Severe

14. When assigning subjective pain severity to numbers, which one correlates with moderate?

   a. 1

   b. 2

   c. 3

   d. 4

   e. 5

15. When using the standard system used by Medical Evaluators to determine the frequency that patients experience symptoms, which percentage best describes "intermittently?"

    a. Approximately 25% of the time

    b. Approximately 50% of the time

    c. Approximately 75% of the time

    d. Whatever duration the patient feels like it's happening

16. The duration of how long an occurrence lasts can be measured in seconds, minutes, hours, days, etc.

    True or False

17. Which of the following are important aspects to note about a client's pain?

    a. Severity

    b. Quality

    c. Duration

    d. If it radiates

    e. All of these

18. The term "ADL's" refers to:

a. A type of stretching technique

b. Attention Deficit List

c. Acute Dental Lesion

d. Activities of Daily Living

19. Your SOAP notes should focus on clients':

a. Dream descriptions

b. Hobbies

c. Special needs

d. Chief complaints

20. Objective complaints are those which can typically be _____ by the examiner.

a. Understood

b. Imagined

c. Measured

d. Ignored

21. Information elicited by using your visual and palpatory skills is considered a valid objective finding in the medical world.

   True or False

22. Regarding significant negative findings:

   a. It's good to let the client express them, but there's no need to document them.

   b. They should not be taken seriously since they are not "positive" findings.

   c. Clients often report them, but they are not important.

   d. They can be important objective findings.

23. Noting both positive and negative findings:

   a. Is not important.

   b. Only positive findings are important.

   c. Provides a bigger picture than only knowing the positive findings.

   d. Is a waste of time and paper.

24. Which are important positive findings to measure and monitor:

   a. Tight soft tissue tone

   b. Inflammation

   c. Positive ROM Findings

   d. All of the above

25. A client's response to palpation, such as pain being elicited, can be considered a valuable *objective* finding.

True or False

26. Your "assessment" of a client can best be described as:

a. Your assessment of their personality and character.

b. What their assets and talents are.

c. Whether or not they will become a good client.

d. Your interpretation, formed opinions and clinical impressions about a client's health status, particularly their chief complaints.

27. Massage therapist are assessing problems mostly for the purpose of:

a. Deriving a diagnosis.

b. To show empathy.

c. To help form clinical impressions.

d. To impress clients.

28. You do not need to describe the exact positive objective findings in detail when writing them in your assessments.

True or False

Learn more ways to advance your professional skills and practice success at MastersInMassage.com

29. If a client reports they are feeling worse or not improving, it's best to not mention this in your SOAP notes.

    True or False

30. Generally speaking, if a client's chief complaint continues to plateau or worsen, it may be best to:

    a. Ignore it and hope for the best.

    b. Give them positive affirmations.

    c. Give them a free or discounted session.

    d. Refer them out for further evaluation.

31. Your "Plan" should do which of the following?

    a. Describe the plan of action you plan to take to manage a client's care.

    b. Be based on all clinical impressions derived from the important information you have gathered about a client.

    c. Describe your treatment goals.

    d. All of these.

32. It's important to assure clients that you will absolutely be able to correct their postural abnormalities and align their structure.

    True of False

33. If you have ever helped a client's scoliosis or other condition, it's alright to assure other clients who have the same problem that you can correct theirs too.

True or False

34. It's reasonable to explain to clients who present *without* a permanent condition, that they may receive some degree of improvement.

True or False

35. The best way to manage your clients' care is by doing what:

a. Let them come and go as they please without making any recommendations.

b. Just sign them up for discounted packages of care.

c. Suggest Programs of Care where you measure and monitor their progress.

36. It's important to write in your SOAP notes the self-care strategies that you suggest to clients.

True or False

37. It's fine to explain a self-care strategy to a client, but let them do it however they like, even if it's wrong, to avoid embarrassing them.

True or False

 Learn more ways to advance your professional skills and practice success at MastersInMassage.com

38. A popular self-care strategy mnemonic is having clients take their ____.

    a. BEDS

    b. REDS

    c. MEDS

    d. NSAIDS

39. If a client expresses to you that they have confusion or complaints about a self-care strategy that another practitioner suggested to them, it's best to:

    a. Tell them not to do it.

    b. Suggest they call the practitioner and tell them.

    c. Possibly suggest one that you feel might work better.

    d. b and c

40. In addition to SOAP notes helping you better manage your clients' care, when clients recognize that you keep SOAP notes, it increases their respect, credibility and professional perceptions of you.

True or False

Learn more ways to advance your professional skills and practice success at MastersInMassage.com

Test Question Answers

1. F	21. T
2. F	22. d
3. T	23. c
4. a	24. d
5. T	25. T
6. e	26. d
7. F	27. c
8. d	28. T
9. d	29. F
10. b	30. d
11. d	31. F
12. a	32. F
13. b	33. T
14. c	34. T
15. b	35. c
16. T	36. T
17. e	37. F
18. d	38. c
19. d	39. b
20. c	40. T

Made in the USA
Columbia, SC
17 July 2021